Eastern Sunsets Beneath Western Skies

Eastern Sunsets Beneath Western Skies

ISBN 978-1-304-07267-2

Published at https://www.lulu.com

All media links available @linktr.ee/jamiehester

Eastern Sunsets Beneath Western Skies

by

Jamie Hester

Contents

Womb 1
Alien 2
Amidst the Speed of a Moment 3
Candlelight 4
That Which Is in a Name 5
Casper 6
Pack 7
The Corner Window on Main 8
Saturday Morning Cartoons 9
Windowpane 10
There Remained 11
There's No Going Back 12
Kingdom Come 13
Nightmares and Daydreams 14
Origins 16
Coping With Today 17
The Air Is Ocean 18
Pyro 20
Relic 21
Born of Dreams 22
Tin Man 23
Breakdown 24

Setting Suns 26
Mirror 27
The Edge of Inspiration 29
Muse 30
Quiet Hours 31
Unanswered Echoes 32
The Labyrinth Within 33
All the Fish in the Sea 34
Life's Piercing of Love's Dream 36
The Bullet Casings of Elysium 37
Impressions of a Shadow 38
Salve 39
As I Search for Sleep 40
Dance 41
The Weight of a Pen 42
Flowers 44
Bouquet 45
Unconditional 46
Lazarus 47
Building Yesterday 49
The Apparitions of Reflection 50
The Dust of Dreams 52
Life of Shadows 53
Etched of Rain 54

Soliloquies 55
Portraits 56
I Am 58
Puzzles 59
Mortal Hands 60
Cirque De La Lune 61
Rat Race 62
Martyrs 63
Static Daydream 64
Wanderlust 65
Islands 66
Are You Listening? 68
Starlit Waters 70
Bearing Gifts 72
Et Tu? 73
Sandcastles 74
Liar 76
Depths 78
Home Movies 79
Lines Within Illusions 80
Vacancies 81
By Any Other Name 83
Wish 84
Echoes Amongst the Rain 85

Watershed 86
The Strength Within a Tear 87
Here and There 89
Reflection 90
Descending 92
Not To Wonder 93
Dreaming To Fly 94
Starlight 95
Meditation 96
Inside Out 97
Scribe 98
Profane 99
The World Still Lingers 100
Western Horizons 101
Reverse Horizons 102
Four Stops ‘til Home 104
Within the Fading Light 107

Womb

Scrape away the scabs.
Note not a single bruise.
Pull the heart from its frame.
Wipe away every salty drop.
Dilute any impulse or thought
back to the unremembered.
Remove every stroke marked
by the brush of life's hand.
See before sight.
Listen before sound.
Trace back every line to before it begins.
If only I could re-immerse my soul in some embryonic sea
and unravel the sinews that crisscrossed buried chambers
as time whispered through the harvest leaves.

Alien

I wish I could remember birth,
only to remember how it must have felt.
Those days long faded,
yet I think I still know.
You emerge into some foreign world,
away from everything that made sense.
You stare at all those unknown faces.
I know because
nothing ever came to make sense.
I know because
I still see those faces
etched frozen as time flows around.

I wonder when that moment was that I first
peered into a reflection as if I saw someone else.
I still wonder at that reflection
still staring back within myself.
I still wonder who that is
from someplace else.

Amidst the Speed of a Moment

Amidst the speed of a moment,
within a darkness of lights,
it still flashes in that place all my own…
In sickness back to health,
over the drone of steel,
within a faceless crowd,
in my weakness,
through a looking glass of liquid salt,
within the arms of a crimson well…
the depths of which I've never seen…

Amidst the speed of a moment,
in the flicker of eternal seconds,
within a passing scene reflected…
imposed over the flow of fleeting portraits…
Within concrete arteries entombed beneath forgotten lights,
within a sprawling darkness encasing a crowd of two,
through the frailty of flesh,
within an embrace of rust…

Amidst the speed of a moment…
I remember still.

Candlelight

Shadows grew amongst the candlelight
I don't quite remember when.
The sugar etching in the candlelight still mattered to someone,
before something broke within.
Somehow song turned to echoes
and time slipped away again.
I could blame imagined angels
and all the powder exhaled from blackened lungs,
but perhaps the pyres were only symptoms of the mismatched
edges untethered by the shards.
Wings were never fitting
once daydreams faded away.
I could blame the silent kings
that etched the stones
atop these unfilled graves,
but the crownless prince was never buried
only left amongst the bones laced with clay.
With a final breath the lines and faces fade,
and the shadows still remain.

That Which Is in a Name

In the search for significance a little boy once found a name.
He treasured every letter, every syllable of the same.
This was not branded, not given by them.
It was passed down in blood, kin upon kin,
all the more cherished for the uncrowned of many names.
It was his hearts hope, his all alone.
So, it was with the name under which he grew,
the only bit of meaning he ever really knew.
He climbed family trees, secure in the shade of their branches.
He smiled bittersweet smiles and looked down from the heights.

Did this little boy love such a thing for itself?
Did he love it for its sound, its structure, or something else?
Was there some grand history which he made live on?
Maybe the treasure was to be named at all.
Then again maybe the significance
was never in the name at all.

Casper

Have you ever felt like your souls on fire,
yet there's not enough light…
that darkness becomes you
despite the stars so bright?
Maybe there is no soul to speak of,
or maybe I've just been losing the fight.
Maybe I slipped trying to hold on through the cold and the rain,
Don Quixote only imagining the dream and reality all the same.
The thinnest shell of pretense whispers with the cadence of
weighted bone.
I never cared for reindeer games or the emptiness they've sold.

Time after time I find myself here again,
my only solace an empty page to fill,
and a pen my only friend.
I gaze upon the tagged gray walls
only my inner eye seems to see.
I am the mistranslation
of someone else's dream,
foundering in the questions
of every breath I concede.
With the precipice of every syllable,
I leap just one more time,
but no matter how many lines,
I only return to the same crumpled pages
and warm my hands against those embers…
unformed words burning every synapse of an overactive mind.
There is no peace beyond those borders,
no peace within this place…
only the daydream of a Casper that never left a trace.

Pack

The pack encloses.
He peers through the storm.
In desperation he searches.
No friendly faces dwell.
Suddenly the world spins…
razor haze all around.
Scavenging eyes stare voraciously
through the mingling of raindrops and blood.
The world disperses.
There in that mountain,
blissfully or cursed,
the wolf shade wanders, has wandered,
since the seconds eon of dusk all alone.
The moonlit eyes always stare.
The serrated smiles always tear.

The Corner Window on Main

Come, come all gather ‘round.
Isn’t that funny? Oh yes, quite so,
that out of place figure over there,
the one in the corner to the right?
Now, now no need to fight.
Yes, that odd one in the corner,
that quiet one over there.
Yes, yes; why such notice?
Such a waste of attention you’ve spent.
But if we clear those scratches,
clean just a bit of that dirt…
No, no; too many scratches,
too many, and too deep.
Besides, its eyes are all blurry,
is that a smudge on its cheek?
Yes, yes it looks like a blush,
perhaps just the remnant of an errant smear…
even funnier, how funny,
so shadowed a thing.
Laugh louder, laugh all around.
Look dear, look;
there’s even a slight frown.
Oh quite, or is that a grimace?
How funny, how funny.
Laugh louder, laugh louder;
come, come laugh all around.
Come now, let’s not tarry,
there’s nothing here that profound,
just a dusty old patchwork
misplaced from the lost and found.
Let us carry on,
the shadows are deepening,
with the sun going down.
No sense in wasting the daylight
upon something so unsound.

Saturday Morning Cartoons

Imagine if you could walk on air as long as you didn't look down.
Imagine that dogs and cats could talk, that elephants could fly.
What if cars could drive themselves and planes knew how to land?
What if appliances could go off on adventures of their own?

Imagine that you could walk on water as long as you kept looking straight ahead.
Imagine that birds didn't always fly south.
What if a dog could be a mouse's best friend?

Imagine that you could run through the tunnel a coyote painted on a rock.
Imagine that you could stop yourself in mid fall.
What if chipmunks could form a band?
What if the moon was really cheese?

Imagine life a Saturday Morning Cartoon.
What if one could just simply laugh away the pain?

Windowpane

He's been looking out that window
through a pane only he can see.
He's been looking up from the hollow ground asking,
why did you bury me?
The toughest thing about tough love
are all the echoes in the deep,
the screams held within a plasma furnace,
against the clank of tin and the silence in between.
The boy has been waiting in that shell of a house,
the shade of seasons passed,
and dreams that used to be.
Of course, that shell could be mere illusion
and that boy within that calcified house only a fitful dream.
He's persisted so quietly year after year
and so I sit with him on occasion, every now and then,
and find myself within these lines again.
Amidst the deaths of winter and the births of spring,
through the summer's heat and the gently falling leaves…
I've seen those haunted eyes staring right through me.
He sits there still with every stroke,
still asking where you've been.

There Remained

There in that picture was the flesh and blood that used to be,
and yet… that little boy in that picture, that isn't me.
I see a man I have known…
No, on second thought…
I probably never really knew that man there within those edges.
Did I ever really know him at all?
All that was between them … if ever there was,
is washed in the wake of time and separated by the unsaid.
I can't blame that stranger alone for everything beyond those
borders of white.
I can only regret those things never said.
I exist outside of that frame, though I can never help wondering
every time I passed that captured moment,
before the years stretched to memories,
if with some secret words that boy could have stayed.
They could have reached out their hands
and within that picture remained.

There’s No Going Back

There’s a picture on a wall
among another’s memories arrayed.
A boy stands in some frozen sunlight,
next to perpetual shade,
below a tree I still pass every day.
I want to stand in that same place,
that same place in that same time,

but there’s no going back.

I want to tell him all the things we may come to know,
all that we came to know. I would tell him…
I’m not sure.
What do you tell the boy you can’t remember you were?

But there’s no going back anymore…

Kingdom Come

A figure sits in the shadows upon a throne of thorns.
His jagged face shines with the streams of passions he has borne.
He sits in the soul chilling shadows…
a relic of something that once believed
in the reality of sunbeams and the mosaic of autumn leaves.
Phantoms of elsewhere burn in his eyes.
A spirit was left alone against the salted tides,
to drown in a lovely darkness…
to weep a melancholy hatred…
to give birth to something perhaps before only latent,
within sandstone labyrinths and smiles so carefully painted.

A kingdom was abandoned,
left to the dreamless,
left to the pack,
and to the serpent's lore.
It was within the infinite space
confined in the finite of a time and a place,
on this side of that door,
the undeclared prince found the only peace
he would come to know anymore.

A kingdom was gained.
The land lay blanketed in the gray of ash.
The skies flashed among the shadows
as the storm clouds slowly passed.
Raindrops fell steadily, heavily upon the ground,
where dark pools converged upon the mountainside,
only to fall into valleys and drown in the sea.

A single tear escapes the gaze of a taut face.
A weary head drops to rest in pale hands.
He returns to his blanket of solitude.
His distant eyes turn to slits
as he sinks into an uneasy rest once more.

Nightmares and Daydreams

Beyond icy crowns and crimson haze,
through valleys deep,
with lasting gaze
upon stars that have shown between passing grays…
Beyond snowcapped teeth,
born of frost giants and feral things…
within blackened wood,
beneath a fleeting moon…
a cloaked shadow casts
his gaze at last upon the darkened waters
and with anxious grasp upon a wooden staff
stirs ripples into portent dreaming.

The uncrowned prince stands upon the threshold of his daydream solace once more.
From the portal of the finite will emerge the herald of waking,
the serpent born of diurnal tides.
The red eyes pierce his being… those eyes that haunt.
This scourge of haven ever rises, to remind the child within the walls
of the lands he'd wandered with the prince
before the dreaming birthed these halls.

Within the ripples of the waters, the cloaked shadow sees the first head dive.
Its fangs draw the icy blood that molds his heart.
The second head slithers down to rip his lungs apart.
The putrid scaly heads writhe and twist in their never-ending exultation.
Once more fear grips his core.
Once more he must decide between flight or the sword.
The ugly serpent's heads stare at his exposed soul and savagely grin.
He curses his weaknesses without and within.
Tears stream down alabaster skin as his resolve withers before his demons risen again.

Hisses and laughter threaten to drown out the thunder of his night.
Despair threatens to overcome him as a rush of blood takes his sight.
Doubt undercuts his balance as gravity bends his knee.

Beneath barren crest, shallow breath from chest heaves
as a rumble builds within the skies across which the stars had once shined.
Lightning laces the sky and finds a kindred spark
within the gaze of the prince's tired eyes.
Flames spring forth and spread,
consuming the scars and the flesh weighing spirits unwed.
Pieces burn away to reveal the crumbled turrets beneath.
The serpent sees itself reflected, torn skin from bone.
Finally, the uncrowned prince finds the strength to stand.
He rises with incandescent sword in hand.
It is his turn to truly grin.
Stumbling backward the serpent finds nothing but space where a portal had just been.

The prince's blade plunges into its life stream and tears into its chest.
Never again shall this serpent of that hell cross thresholds wept of coral years.
Its warm green blood cakes his arms and drops from burning steel.
At his feet lay severed its heads…

The water stills as the ripples slowly pass.
The cloaked shadow leans once more on twisted staff.
He glances at the moon retreating behind advancing clouds only lined by the light is casts.
He wanders among the deeper shadows within the forest once again.

Origins

A boy would sit inside of the battlements,
within his own fortress walls,
made of salts, of resins,
made of borders bound by silent halls.
He would sit, enthralled
with worlds only of imagination,
within the quiet places once plagued,
with the absence, the unspoken, and all the bottled rage.
Learning the possibilities of words gave the spark to a flame.
His imagination raged through the forests of his mind.
Waking began to fade to daydreams in the smoke of the ashes.
Anger just became thunder rumbling within the wind,
sorrow merely rivers cutting through the caverns within.
The shores stretched beyond sight,
despite the threshold cocoon of skin.
On that island, within the depths,
the uncrowned prince was born
and ever after remained.

Coping With Today

Lost in a wake of shadows
coping with today.
I clutch my twisted stomach,
sit and hold my swimming head.
I dream delusional clarities
until the precarious tides of the inexpressible
overtake me once again.

The Air Is Ocean

I've never played *The Floor Is Lava,*
but I've played *The Air Is Ocean.*
I've played it ever since somewhere
between memory and the rainbow roulette of pills.
It's a game of chicken,
body versus mind,
where winning feels like survival
and survival plays with time.
The value of each breath
adds resonance to the pleas echoing inside,
telling your lungs to breathe…

Just breathe…

Breathe through the stale claustrophobia
of the people caving in…
of the walls eroding before the surge
of the growing silent din.

Just breathe…

Breathe through that old familiar feeling,
like you're speaking with an old familiar friend…

Just breathe…

Breathe through the distilled exhalations
when the oxygen seems paper-thin,
when the pains begin again…
that constriction the doctors called anxiety
that lets the waters in…
these phantom heart attacks
the doctors told me were just the jester's grin.

Just breathe…
Just try to breathe again…

It's just a friendly reminder you're never far
from where you've been.
Just breathe in rhythm with the descending lines
from left to right again.

Pyro

I burn through pages
like wildfire through trees
each syllable contagious,
spread by every line conceived.

Relic

I stare into the frozen light at the face of a boy that time once knew.
I search through the eyes reflected upon myself within that altered light.
There was everything. There was anything.
There was held forgotten and future memories we only wish I knew.
That child, that boy, frozen in light…
Within the depths of those irises were held dreams, now so long undreamt.
Saltwater washes the relic light of daydreams lost.

Born of Dreams

If only you could've mended a broken heart
as easily as a frame,
filled it with something more
than that with which it came.
He's seen you fix the broken
with nails, with hammer, with such carefully crafted aim…
but those were only objects
of measured weight and string.
If only you had known how to stitch a splintered spirit
before you gave the thought a name.
Perhaps you should've seen
beyond your preconceptions
when you birthed a shadowed life from dreams.
Perhaps you should have given thought
before you spoke of spreading wings.
I wish I had never read the tale
scripted in between.

Tin Man

All those attributes of a metallic man…
The firmness of iron…
The solid demeanor
would only shield.
It too could be weathered and changed by time,
but longer it stands
and stronger it holds.
With a can of oil rain can still fall.
Does he not have sight,
can he not reach out and grasp?
Can he not speak his mind?
Why ask for a heart?

Breakdown

You never asked how I felt,
what I dreamed,
what I feared.
You never wondered what I thought,
you just went about your day.
You only spoke in silence
and in the silence, I learned how not to be okay.
We all face the world,
but I always felt I faced the world alone.
The silence introduced me to that,
wrapped me in that,
froze my breath in that alone.
I found a salve in writing echoes never spoken
among the decaying walls.
I tried to make the alone okay,
but the silence always lingered,
as every summer changed to fall.
It always lingers still,
regardless of the sunshine or the rain.
I still try to write away the echoes,
try to make the syllables match the cadence,
to make the ringing speak.
Maybe it's the naivete of some inner child
thinking that they could somehow write the silence away.
Maybe some part of them
just always hoped that even if only written,
the echoes could escape the walls
into the ether and finally find their way.
You never asked me how I felt,
what I dreamed, what I feared.
You never asked me what I thought,
what I loved,
you never asked me about my pain.
You just spoke in sharpened jests
and went about your day.
You only ever truly spoke in silence

and in the silence, I learned how to live with
all the echoes of not okay.

Setting Suns

I just wanted something,
something he never quite knew how to ask.
We wanted something he was shamed to mask.
Maybe in the end all we ever really wanted,
just for once, was to not to feel this feeling,
this something between me and you.
I know the boy you once saw before you
was not your favorite son.
I know because he told me so.
He's been right here within your gaze
with every setting sun.
He tells me with every ache held inside
and every tear drop shed.
Your son has told me all my life it seems
of the love of a father
for the son he'd never see,
somewhere in that something
between the you and me.

Mirror

Mirror vestige…
My shackled friend,
when all else fades,
there are none left
but your reflection
as each night overtakes each day.
If I was strong
I could've stood and faced…
If I was stronger…
I could've chased the shadows away.

Muted refraction,
my ghost that only I can see…
You who have followed my steps
through every stitch and dream…
I've dreamt of many things
I barely remember the dreaming of anymore.
I've feasted on poisoned apples.
I've laid to rest almost hoping
not to see waking anymore.

My shadowed impression…
I've chipped away the make up
behind the creak of every door,
only to find
the gloss beneath the lines not so upside down,
where hinges were before.
I've heard that we live life after life
upon this world until we get it right.
Perhaps just one more time and I could fix
all these things that mar the reflection
I see when the twilight bends your light.
I could lift the weight,
choking the whispers from your breath.
I could heal the scars,
cut with sharpened syllables…

cut with hostile breath.
I could heal the bruises.
I could stay our hand.
Perhaps just one more time
and I could…
Just one more time
and I could do more than
just dream of beginnings once again.

The Edge of Inspiration

The sword of inspiration is a sharp double edge.
I write verses like track marks,
part of me living in the suffering,
only sparking in the suffering,
the other trying to extinguish the flame.

Muse

My voracious companions, my misbegotten twins,
I know not where one shade ends and the other begins,
nor if the difference is all mere illusion in the end.
I just know the pit in my stomach that aches when you feed.
I shake with the whisper of your voices.
Your grip, my steadfast muses,
brings a halt to my plodding steps
and brings ground to knees.

Quiet Hours

It's in the quiet hours
the reel always runs,
spinning through
my eyes like a loaded gun.
There's no end
to the tempo,
of the rattle and the hum,
of daydream visions
and realities never gone.

Unanswered Echoes

Sing to me my soul of those receding waters, the forgotten cradle.
Scream out those mysteries locked indecipherably within.
There's a gnawing with no beginning and no end,
the illusion of an answer to a question
I have still to find the words or the direction in which to ask.
I only stumble over verses, cursing dead ends,
only finding myself with each progressive grain
listless just the same.

The Labyrinth Within

The prince weeps at his realm,
since time before memory in crumbling disarray.
The jester laughs, thin lips parted,
exhaling bitterness and cynicism with each breath.
The general is called to arms too late,
on all sides beset…
by his own, by the king… the jester…
by whispers and unrest…

The beast of reflection,
that dark matter birthed within the mystery of being,
scratches and claws at the labyrinth within,
as each play their part
and the drumbeat begins.

All the Fish in the Sea

All the cliches
they all throw back at me/
mean nothing to a heart
treading the sea/
where the fish are all sharks
and I can't help but bleed/
with all the gashes
your lips cut into the very heart of me/
not from kisses
but from words that you speak/
I thought I was living
but now I see/
I'm waking up from make believe/
make believe that love exists
and that there's someone for me/
make believe in miracles
and what's meant to be/
when all I ever wanted
was to never wake from these dreams/
never see past the stars/
never drop to my knees/
never remember the needle/
the bittersweet suture
it's all too uneasy to see/
but so easy to batter
to bruise and to bleed/
I don't want all your wishes
your pats or your pleas/
to just see the clouds with the linings
that don't look so silver to me/
just an overcast sky
raining teardrops like me/
I just see all that you wanted
versus all that I am/
all that I ever wanted
versus the seconds I've had/

to pretend to cherish a feeling
cut away by the sands/
drowned out by the sea
of the comfortless cliches/
like all these words laid to rest on pages
that are all just pale reflections in the end/
the fish are all sharks
and all they want is to feed/
to leave nothing left
but the ghost of a dream.

Life's Piercing of Love's Dream

Eros how cursed is your joke
played upon a daydream fool,
how damnable your poisoned arrows
that turn love's words to ashes
and pierce a tender breast,
a mirage of crystal waters
turned to sand,
swallowed by a soul
with nothing left to bare
but the affliction in the mirror
at whom it's left to stare.
Those scars beneath the painted mask
I've traced with trembling hands
and washed away with stinging tears
in the silence of a soul
too broken to ever share.
I spit upon the punctures
these errant marks have left
and wear each scar with the knowledge
your power all but myth.
I'd rip the wings from off your back
if ever I hoped again to rise.
I'd stab the very sight from each of your cherubic eyes
if only to prove love blind.
I'd impale this tattered paper heart upon a thousand arrows
if only to bleed into the numbness
that is all there is to dream.

The Bullet Casings of Elysium

I’ve traveled many miles in these shoes
just to petrify a moving heart unmoved,
amber encased and fossilized through.
The bullet casings still litter
the battlefield of hearts consumed.
In this land of Elysium,
battered and bruised…
this tourniquet of tomorrow
doesn’t treat the ghosts of yesterday
nor the quiet rattle of the bones
scattered along the way.

Impressions of a Shadow

My lust…
My love…
My passion…
My vice…
You were everything when I had nothing,
both darkness and light.
Do you think of me when you regret (reminisce…)?
Do you think of me at all?
If I had all those years back
that I once wished not at all,
would you still wish to have been there despite the fall?
There remains an aching impression of a shadow
I still wonder I dreamed at all.

Salve

To know love is to see the sweetest
dreams awaken to falling sands,
your breath clutching your chest with white knuckles,
while memory grasps at today
with the weight of open hands.
The most beautiful petals
always fade to the darkest hues
just before the thorns cut,
but the rain never cleanses the wound.
Love is the mirage of a soldier
daydreaming through war,
waking up to reality with new scars to tend.
Love is mind and breath playing roulette
with your heart on a string.
This is the last time I cast a bottle to the sea,
the last bit of salt
I ever plan to seed.
Cupid's arrows are poisoned
so, I turn restless again
to the shelter of these words.

As I Search for Sleep

These things that stir,
began to stir,
as I lay down to rest…
I wonder what you're doing when you wake,
what you dream when you drift to dreaming.
When I think of you
I can't help but wonder
if you're thinking of me too.
How as I lay my head down,
you follow me to sleep.

Dance

Have you seen the place where angels dance,
a place still lived in dreams?
It's somewhere past that gray,
perhaps just beyond the trees.

See the dim shine of the lost,
of what fell along the way.
See it in the river's flow
whose sound makes restless nights.
Feel it in the song still playing since the dawn of day.

Remembrance comes in the dream still dreamt,
of a place so long ago,
where time stood still,
where angels danced,
somewhere in the gray, just beyond the trees.

The Weight of a Pen

I'm at that point,
no use denying it's true,
wonderin' if you're thinking of me
as I'm thinkin' of you.
I feel something igniting,
all my daydreams attest.
I'm fightin' to focus,
so I bear deep on the lines,
all bottomed out bottles
that pump ink into rhyme.
My heart starts counting the time
'til the next time you speak,
the next time you smile.
I just need the words
to release all these feelings
all dying to speak,
all the embers you've stoked
that are burning the seams
of the patchwork I stitched
with flightless wings.
I hope you don't think it too much.
I'm just being me.
I've never known any other way,
least not that was me,
this heart in my chest tattooed on my sleeve.
My poetry has always been
my only release,
since before I can remember,
since before all the seams,
just searchin' for
the threads that might save
the stuff of dreams.
All these words have been the blueprint
for the few who've cared to see
the truths that lie behind the static
of melanin screens.

I just write to make the weight of this heart
match the weight of this pen.

Flowers

I'm normally so good at putting this heart to this pen
but equilibrium's fickle in the state that I'm in.
Take a deep breath... upon exhale I'll figure out just where to begin.
Paper was always my fortress, my walls, and my friend.
My heartbeat's defined each syllable
of all the things that I've been.
My towering opus
laid bare in plain sight,
but the hieroglyphic static sounds an enigmatic symphony
as the indifferent world spins.
I just don my headphones and reload my pen.
I measure infinite concepts
with these measured finite lines,
like that secret word
that ushered forth space and time.
I'm just trying to make sense of the daze,
shed light through the haze.
The truth of it is,
I think of you.
I think of you between the stars and the light.
I know that it shows.
My heart's been this worn on my sleeve
since I discovered poetry over prose.
I could wrap a bouquet,
pick the most perfect ones for hours,
but the truth of it is,
these words are my sincerest flowers.

Bouquet

Roses shaded red,
violets dyed blue…
by any other name just as sweet…
until the thorns pierce through.

Unconditional

When someone asks,
‘Do you love me?’,
what they really mean
is ‘Do you love me for now’.
They mean before the us
returns to you and I
and time steals the now.
They mean before each
starlight whisper turns to echoes
and all the lines begin to blur
between the smiles and the frowns.
I am Cain walking with the bayonet heart
of a Father's winged wars,
exhaling the smoke
of all the things
that I imagined we were
until somewhere along the road
I’ve forgotten what tomorrow was for.
Another shot to the heart
just to add to the trail
of spent casings fallen
inert to the floor.
Promises of forever
are just a duel of Russian roulette,
without knowing the paces,
without counting the steps.
It’s a game of not knowing
when the chamber will call the bluff
of promises unbroken
and souls left unrent.

Lazarus

I spent my whole life in love
with a bottle and a pen.
It's funny how the notes
repeat like the lines running thin…
with each crumbled heart,
back to the wide ruled canvas again…
each line inspired
from start 'til the end,
each love a life
to play Lazarus again.

I spent my whole life
in love with the pen,
dueled every demon
and sliced every grin.
I've written through the bullets
and bled through every breath,
seized upon the notes
echoing within my chest.
You think you know the picture
because you picked the frame.
Frames are all illusion
and you barely know my name.

I feel a lot of weight
as the sun goes down.
My heart runs empty
with all the corners I've found,
riddles tucked away
like smiles to a frown…
just another sun set
upon another town
laced with the beats
of that same heartbreak sound.

I watch the shadows
creep along the edges
as the jeweled curtain comes down,
needle to the record
as the heart goes round.
Life flows to the groove
of this infinite sound.
My pocket's been empty
since the last wish was drowned.

I spent my whole life in love
with a bottle and a pen.
It's funny how the notes
repeat like the lines running thin…
with each crumbled heart,
back to the wide ruled canvas again…
each line inspired
from start 'til the end,
each love a life
to play Lazarus again.

Building Yesterday

I thought to build a solid foundation,
as solid as the seemingly ageless stone,
but stone erodes to dust
before the wind and the rain,
to scatter among the currents
inexorably lost among the dunes of memory,
building the deserts of yesterday.
I walk there after the sunset,
footsteps drifting away.
no trace of passing ever remains
but the cold starlight out of reach,
yet haunting my wayward dreams.
Yesterday and tomorrow
are the thorns that mar the present,
bleeding upon the petals,
within the flowering of this haze.
I can never shake the echoes
or the clouds that bring the rain.

The Apparitions of Reflection

This apparition of sentience gets lost in the depths of the morning
sinking somehow between the reflections and all those
forgotten bits of the spectrum each hand takes away.
I daily dance with the skeletons quarantined within my soul,
someplace where angels used to dance
where some dreams, left unengraved,
were laid beneath the weight of stones.
There's a haunting in the ocular window,
stuck somewhere between all the landscapes born of dragons
and all the things touched, tasted, and all the sunsets seen.
So many skylines faded where the currents weave
among the ancient, salted tides.
Though they may have drifted through distances of space and time,
their currents never drifted beyond that dune upon the eastern sands.
Is it just the human condition to be left haunted with the inexorability of time?
Is the world spinning indifferently through the space between the stars,
a ghost light only etching the entropy of their reflections…
for only fleeting moments enshrined?

The chaos of the stitch work started long ago
made the amalgam of the masks
that was the prince and the jester and all the things in between.
Yet these facades of consciousness
were never the soul of the reflection
lost between that mirror and all the things seen.
The truths of the undercurrents
bleed through the echoes
made visible through the hieroglyphs of misspent words.
It is in the solitude of reflections,
somewhere beyond mirrors of glass,
that the truth is stretched across the satyrs and the fairies.

It is stretched across the bones of imagined wings the cratered seas could never hide.

The Dust of Dreams

What do you do when all the comforts
of your life become a briar patch amidst a world of thorns,
all the more stinging for the tender places so exposed
to the elements and the cold.
I wish you could see with your own eyes momma, but you went away.
All foundations have finally crumbled
and your life's work has gone astray.
The maelstrom was seeded from a nexus born of pride, sorrow, and of rage,
where silent walls begat the uncrowned prince,
where unspoken echoes scarred the trace of anything left remembered of some imagined place.
The king and queen must once have spoken of battlements and saving walls of grace.
What seer would've known the poisons therein laced?
Sometimes the unsaid cuts deeper than the edges of a voice.
Sometimes words are better left to choice.
Past down was the unspoken
that twisted and choked the labored echoes that faded to the hall's last breath,
until the realm had fallen
and each heir to dust was left.
May every piercing thorn tear my flesh
for hearts are only pain.
May every raindrop wash away
the lingering that remains.
Maybe I was just always too sensitive for the thorns and the rain,
but at least I had an oasis and an angel instead of this grave.
I etch upon its tombstone with chisel everyday…
as catharsis… as testament…
as something more than…

Life of Shadows

I've lived a life of shadows
with just a pocket full of dreams.
My soul's a ghost town
populated by rumored hauntings
and imaginary friends.
I've woven my webs of symmetry
since my hand first held a pen,
wandering roads traveled
from the beginning to the end.
I've long since bit the fabric of reality
with a jester's grin,
a prince apart from kingdoms
but for the voices in his head,
the stones inside his chest,
and all the shadows that he's wed.
A pariah in a crowd
all rotting from within.
This ghost town speaks
in the whispered creaks
of every rusted hinge
to doors untouched but by
the passing wind.

Etched of Rain

When I was young, I used to love the rain…
the skies blanketed bleak, the whisper of the heralding breeze,
a prince felt more comfortable, more at home, in that world.
The boy, he pretended that those drops were his tears unreleased,
soaking reality, like the soil, with the well hidden beneath…
wandering amidst the growing tides, wandering between two worlds…
under the nexus of the fiery twilight.

Still the rain brings a slight grin.
Still the prince wanders every now and then.
He can still be felt in those drops, his heart heard in the rhythm of the splashing.
His face can still be seen reflected deep within those rippling puddles left atop the concrete plains.

Soliloquies

Birth is the first soliloquy.
Life is just moments of reiteration,
time just a mirror which reflects
the ghost of anonymity
whose only audience is ourselves.
We are all orators rambling, only imagining the theater of our worlds.
No one else will ever see what we see
because the very nature of perspective
renders us irrevocably islands among fleeting shadows that fret about the stage.
My joys, my solace, my sorrows, my pains, my regrets are forever mine alone.
No one wakes to the same sun nor sleeps beneath the same stars.
They all blend differently within the cauldron of our souls,
born into a world that doesn't know you any better than that newborn knew themselves.
Humanity is so many snowflakes
in a blizzard,
each unique despite the encroaching cold front
and in that demarcation
lost within the storm.
So, before that last horizon,
even held in the firmest grasp,
I can’t help but think how we each cross
that threshold alone.
I can't help but think as birth so is life,
just as is life's last breath.

Portraits

Just before the horizon, a bronze sentinel catches the last hues of twilight.
As the sun fades to stars, moonlit dunes glow
before the darkened brackish waters that commune with the open sea.
The soft sonata of the tides ebb and flow
gives melody to the temperate breeze and disperses amongst the boughs of inland canopies.
Diurnal spectrums cast their kaleidoscopic light
across honeysuckle trumpets and maple trees of red and gold.
36.8529 N, 75.9780 W, where ghosts walk
a living boardwalk and where with whispers my soul's confessed.
That twilight still casts a blanket over swing sets boarded by time,
perhaps by now laid to rest.
Streetlights still glow through the panes of invaded halls.
The road still bends to pass by all the cul-de-sacs we knew as kids.
I still see those pictures on the wall,
if only through a weathered temporal lens.
I still remember sprites held as close
as the sisters that once stood between
a lost child and the borders of a frame.
Like the canvas of a photograph,
each particle of atmosphere catches a moments light.
I still see the faces in those phantom moments.
I still see the streetlights and the glow they cast.
I don't remember when we traded those borders for lines on a map.
I don't remember when entropy stole embrace.

Maybe it's all just the inevitability of the hourglass
and the inextricable tethers that chain us all to time.
I've always thought it a choice rather than a demand.
Are we all just blinded by the blasted glass
etched as the hours grow,
while every moment ever frozen is buried beneath the weight

of every grain of sand?
These phantom portraits of moments,
maybe they were just illusion all along.
Maybe the fantasy of a castle was always nothing more than
a lost boy's desperation,
and a jester's sadistic whim.
Maybe nothing matters but these words in the end.
I'll lay these tomes upon their shelves
and count them among the stories I cherish
each night I lay my head to rest.

I Am

Tattered clothes/
tattered heart/
I am.
Guitar strings/
echoes sing/
I am.
Sky blue canvas/
painted red/
I am.
Daydream tomes/
printed homes/
I am.
Scheming cat/
consoling laugh/
I am.

Puzzles

My sisters were always good at puzzles,
I never felt the same.
It has led me to wonder,
can one know the picture by the pieces
without the benefit of the box with which it came?
If one could glue the finished borders
with just a few missing pieces inside,
would it be a portrait just the same?
I've puzzled at the pieces missing
with so many crafted lines,
trying to find the patterns
in all the things we've left behind.
I'd write these misshapen pieces,
trying to make these edges fit,
without the box, that sanctioned image,
etched from unbroken promises,
and preconceptions only dreamed.
I'll never know what that portrait was.
It was never the one he'd seen.
He grew up in the corner, along edges,
seeking those things within.

Mortal Hands

I am Jacob.
I am Cain.
I wrestle with my soul,
I wander restless all the same…
birthright forsaken,
from a divided home.

I am Joseph…
humbled, yet risen
in the shadow of a desert throne.
I am the jester before the court
who grins through the pain alone.

I am the distressed heart of tattered dreams,
unwoven and restitched with
the trembling of mortal hands.

I am the echo of the strings
as neon twilights fade.

I am the daydreams of forgotten words
written upon the thinnest parchment
and drafted in flowing red.

Cirque De La Lune

The lights reveal a littered, unkempt ground.
The air hangs motionless, letting through every sound.
The people sit upon bleachers.
Everything is still but their eyes.
Hair and clothes are dripping dye.
The sales booths are all boarded, the games aborted.
The animals all sleep restlessly within their cage,
gnashing enamel daggers in their subconscious rage.
All the people sit on cold metal, not a single soul unsettled.
The acrobats are all positioned with the greatest care,
with each bead of sweat all the greater for the heights they cannot bear.
Still, the audience is focused on just a single spot,
within the darkened spaces, just a single dot.
The fire eater tries to remember not to burn himself again.
The escape artist is locked in chains.
The painted jester twists his visage into dramatic lines of laughter,
despite the crowds so densely gathered.
He pats the keys within his pockets and carries on amidst the shadows.
Fixated on the same spot, the people stare with rapt suspense.
They all see the tight rope walker precariously stumbling along.
They never knew he was barely holding on,
holding on to the line between here and gone,
swaying between sanity and madness all along.

Rat Race

The masses shove and push past each other everyday
in a never-ending cycle of 'getting ahead.'
One gets past another only to be passed by again.
The sounds of car horns and shouts
ring all through the day and night,
only to be outdone by gun blasts and blades
and a big neon sign that claims, 'Jesus saves.'
Those trampled on fall under,
only to rise again, to make the first the last
and the last first again and again.

A man rushes past all his loved ones,
his partner and his kids,
to get to a cubicle in an office never his.
He forgets 'I love you', kisses, and hugs
all for a machine that only screams 'never enough'.
He trades the priceless for the material
because 'society has deemed it this way'.

If gods exist, they must weep every day,
for lifetimes are wasted on nothing,
and the things most precious are left to tomorrows and yesterdays.

Martyrs

I've heard some people talk
of that which is beyond time and space.
I've heard of the limits of human perception,
of all the potential that lies untapped.
I've heard of the postulation
of a being unconstrained.
All I've ever known I've seen through these eyes,
heard from these ears,
tasted with this tongue,
felt through this skin.
My reality is intrinsically bound by the evidence of my own perception.
I've heard of oblivion, annihilation,
and the absence of me.
Existence may all be a second's denial
amidst some unfathomable void.
We're all prisoners, you, and I,
of this time and this place.
We're each destined the same,
each of us a martyr to the human race.

Static Daydream

I play with syllables beneath the static
of this weathered skin,
stitched with silver linings
to contain the tides within.

Wanderlust

The being wrapped in rags quietly drifting
through the tunnels and byways of the mind
seeks a certain time, a certain moment,
that in the relentless flow has faded from the day.
Electricity sparks on the rails of
mutable metal and illuminates
the twisting and turning recesses
diving and crisscrossing
in a hyperactive mind.
The slits of vacant white
strain at the shooting stars.
Phantom graffiti flickers on
the thin gray walls.
Echoes can be heard
every now and then.

The figure wanders on
with his tatters rustled
ever so softly by the surreal breeze,
each moment wandering again and again.

Islands

No man's an island…?
I've been an island from the womb
to the reflections I now see.
I've been an island,
ever since memories were dreams,
ever since the last leaf fell from the boughs of dead trees.

No man's an island…?
Perhaps in theory I never was…
not in the company of me.
I just contextualized the voices
and turned me to we.
I just rolled them all into bottles
and cast them to the seven seas.
I've gazed out upon the depths
and have floated beneath the stars.
I've traversed the sands swirling
upon the relentless winds of time,
only to find a certainty more certain
with each step left behind.

No man's an island…?
maybe not every person,
perhaps not every soul,
but I see ghosts adrift everyday
in the tide pools and the shoals.
I was an island before the very first sketch was drafted with a pen,
from that sketch of a family portrait,
she told me was never true…
despite what I felt…
despite all they thought they knew.
I was an island when plainer footsteps
were carried away in the ocean breeze…
when plainer steps breeched thresholds by the sea.
I was an island when a king's paper palace
turned to mausoleums in my mind.

I was an island amidst school yard prisons
and an island amongst rows and rows
of dusty printed tomes.
I've been an island unto we
whatever direction I've roamed.
I think upon the steel currents,
every now and then
and remember the horizons…
from east to west, north to south,
to distant shores and back again.

No man's an island…?
I've been an island all my life,
from cradles unremembered,
to graves defined
with epitaphs of chiseled lore.

Are You Listening?

Momma are you listening?
I still see you there someplace beyond a veil.
I see you in the rarest smile.
I still hear you in a voice
that now only echoes from the setting years.

Momma can you hear me?
I need you to know that I'm still here.
I've known the voices and their whispers,
I know the struggle and the tears.
I see glimpses of you that I remember,
just before my heart breaks
and my momma disappears.

You pray in those lonely hours that they'll all just go away.
You pray in all the lonely hours for just one good day.
I too have seen the twilight that takes your sight,
as I plead with you to stay.

Momma can you hear me?
I need you to know I'm still here.
I've known the voices and their whispers,
I know the struggle and the tears.
I see glimpses of you that I remember,
just before my heart breaks
and my momma disappears.

Stay a little longer momma
I still need you here.
Let me hold you just a little longer momma
before the whispers steal your years,
before the violet steels your fears.
Stay a little longer momma,
your little boy still needs you here.

Momma can you hear me?

I need you to know that I'm still here.
I’ve known the voices and their whispers,
I know the struggle and the tears.
I see those glimpses of you that I remember,
just before my heart breaks
and my momma disappears.

Starlit Waters

I wish I knew you,
perhaps 'knew you better' is better said.
I've so long attempted to decipher
all those woven tapestries
in between metal and bone.
I see those things,
those things of you in me,
by reflection, by habit,
even by those things weighted
in the waters underneath.
I can only sit and wonder
at the threads of you
you left woven into me.
Perhaps knowing more of you
I might better know that something
coiled within the deep.
Perhaps in the end it's self-serving,
but are you purer than this distillation
of Stygian nature and the nurturing of broken trees?
Could I be but the shard of a broken mirror,
reflecting things only your weathered eyes have seen?
It's like I see you from the opposite bank
of some raging creek,
so seemingly simple a crossing
save unspoken steps incomplete.
I so often stared at the reflection
I cast in your eyes,
just to try,
to try to trace the lines of what you see
before the waters rushing by.
I've wondered at the snowcapped peaks of disparity
and at the faintest notes of similarity
carried on the wind.

I’ve seen jagged edges
I don’t know whether to call strong or weak.
I’ve seen a logical construction
encasing the abstracts beneath.
I’ve seen glimpses of you through your eyes,
glimpses of that fluctuating shade
settled on the other side.
I’ve seen glimpses of some piece of me
I may never truly know,
as the silence of so many questions
is carried away along the waters that
under starlight have always flowed.

Bearing Gifts

They accepted my father's gift.
I don't quite remember when I decided it wasn't for me.
I think it was somewhere between the shadows of
the romantic poets and the allure of mythic seas.
They received my father's gift.
In the malignant silence, I've most clearly seen.
They received my father's gift
and now only memories remain of we.
I sometimes wonder if that pronoun ever truly fit
the roots this briar patch came to be.
They have borne my father's gift.
I rejected it when I first put pen to page.
Every time I type a line,
I exorcise the crippling silence
of the walls that untold years have made.
With every single syllable
I deny my father's unspoken gift
and the inheritance of its wake.
It is they who have borne my father's gift.
Its sheath for one is rage.
They scream their silence among the walls
and trample open gates.
The other blunts their silence
with the edge of northern wastes.
They swing without any consideration
for marks their gift will make.
They bear my father's gift.
It lingers in a shell of memory
where gather ghosts untold.
I refuse my father's gift.
I transmute my inheritance with every page I've ever torn
from the tatters of a soul.

Et Tu?

All that love has ever taught me
is that you're just like all the rest,
just another shadow amidst the passersby
that tread the waters of this waking tomb.
I'd bought your truths under still older stars,
amidst the immolation of rotted walls,
amidst the thorns that grew within,
that grew around,
that aging shell of youth.
The mirages laid across the sands of time are but the echoes left of you.
There is no more to your varied visage
than the space between the dying night,
no more than the crumbling of weighted trees of stone.
Perhaps I hadn't seen the shifting sands for the smoke and mirrors of the tide.
Now I see all the faces,
despite the murky waters,
despite the ripples across my own.
You taught me there is no connection
in those tide pools,
just the inevitable erosion of time,
when the last breath evaporates,
and only cavities are left behind.

Sandcastles

Do you remember the tidal waters of newborn lands
where the dreamers birthed their daydreams
within their castles made of sand.
I still remember the fireflies glowing
among the mortal moons and
the Christmas eve wishes whispered
before the dawn of snowless afternoons.
I know not when the walls began to crumble,
if ever they stood at all.
I miss the lost of those sandcastle dreams,
when two sisters had a brother,
and a brother without a family
still imagined resting among the branches
grown of lowland trees.

Even while drifting within a haze of gray,
upon so many ancient seas,
I thought of those newborn shores,
I thought of what I always thought would be.
I'd stare at a starlit expanse just the same
as I drifted among the twilight currents of fathoms deep,
never realizing, perhaps just not believing,
how truly distant those shores had come to be.
All that's left of those sandcastles
lies in hearts too pierced to bleed,
for within the sunset of that newborn shore I lost a piece of me.

With salted eyes I once again set weary step
upon those long remembered shores,
where sandcastles still meet the tides
and become no more.
I sat again upon those same dunes where once I myself had
dreamed.
Yet alas!
I fear there's no return to lands so lost,
no return to boughs of rotted trees.

I returned to find
that all that's left of sandcastles
are hearts too pierced to bleed,
for within the sunset of that newborn shore
I lost a piece of me.

Liar

I see alphanumeric coding
lit among the dimness with a name
I didn't know that I only used to know
before the silence took them from the frame.
The steady barrage retraced those lines
only two of us had known.
It's funny… I don't remember the specific contours,
I just remember the feeling,
a self-portrait of someone else's dream
turned to hauntings,
beneath the weight of stone.
I doubt my only critic even remembers her words that day,
that it wasn't true, this wasn't them,
that somehow, the truth was that other portrait,
the one witnessed by the camera's lens, when mom had fixed our hair.
They were younger then, we were younger still,
yet the ghosts were always there.

With an innocuously green accept,
I hear a voice I may have only thought I'd known,
but I remembered all the same.
I'll always remember that voice.
I'll remember the sharp edge of the words
that cut beneath the surface,
just as every sling and every arrow cast
among this civil fray.
I'll remember those words as part of a chrysalis
from which I was awakening as I watched my mother fade.
I was called a liar. I don't know if I've ever admitted it until this day.
I was a liar, a liar for years untold.

The lie was always in telling myself that that lens' portrait was ever home.
I don't know when I'd convinced myself that that self-sketched portrait wasn't true.
The lie was never in the truth of the broken embrace
I felt within her arms that day,
even though the child in me wept that his mother had gone away.
The lie was never in the fading
I had no choice but to watch within the reflection of her eyes.
It wasn't in the heartbreak of unassailable delusion,
nor in the hallucinations I bore witness to by her side.
It wasn't in the shuddering sobs I watched her inconsolably cry.

They had built rotted walls upon a delusion
and held on past remembering
that there was anything left to hold onto inside.
I am a liar, but her fading, my tears were never the lie.
The lie was to myself,
over all those years gone by.
The lie was that carefully staged portrait
lost to the ravages of time.
Home was just a dream that died with the light in her eyes.

Depths

I thought I'd built a solid foundation,
as solid as the lingering stone,
but stone erodes with the wind and the rain,
to dust,
among the currents to wash away,
deposited inexorably to the depths of memory
far beneath the waves.
I've walked in that Atlantean sunset
where there are no footsteps to fade away,
where relics stand frozen in time,
where all that remains are the haunting currents
of lightless wayward skies.

Home Movies

What is space but an invisible line?
What is time but the space between
two frames within the reel of one's own mind?

Lines Within Illusions

I'm beginning to see the lines my father's seen,
crisscrossing the residual haze of unrealized dreams.
Hands rough, eyes dimmed,
I wish I knew now what I hadn't then.
If only I wasn't so myself
those times I wasn't him.
I think even without words,
maybe through the iterations of hourglass lenses,
I know just a little more of him now…
some amalgamation of translation
beyond the arithmetic mean.
I've seen the light waves ripple and swirl
along the raging creek.
I've seen the lines unmasked by time
as the sands are carried along the bed beneath.
Though the chameleon facade of the undefinable unspoken
never lingers too far from in between.
Sometimes I can almost swear
I hear faint echoes in that void between you and me.

Vacancies

When all that's said and done,
I'll never know what's behind those eyes.
Perhaps there are fallen angels
or better demons
that all just try to hide
behind iris lenses
and the scar tissue of vacant eyes.
I used to want to find a purpose
in the vacancy of those eyes…
something to make the pain meaningful…
something to untwist all the knotted sores inside.
Yet, I discovered a purpose
in every stutter I scratched through every line,
searching through the hazel kaleidoscope of mine.
I may have never mended
but I found something in the fire.
I found something left inside.
The backdraft from the inspiration
has lit so many nights,
haunted by unspoken melodics
that sing among the vacancies
that pierced with every sigh.
I light the spark every time
I stumble across a rhyme,
every time I dream
of the horizon.
I learned to make tracks
with every tear I've ever resigned to all the pages
that have tried to fill the vacancies
I inherited from your eyes.
You don't know me,
though perhaps of late you've tried.
I used to believe I'd level every forest
just to find the paper to draft the answers
to all the questions I always felt inside.
I used to dream of God and wonder why,

why are all the sunsets
as quiet as the darkness in your eyes.
I still warm phantom hearts by the fires.
I still look to the skies.
I still wonder at the dotted canopy
and try to fill the spaces we both hide.
I light the spark every time
I stumble across a rhyme,
every time I dream
of the horizon,
I learned to make tracks
with every tear I've ever resigned to all the pages
that have tried to fill the vacancies
I inherited from your eyes.

By Any Other Name

We all found lines in the sand to bury love beneath,
entombed with platitudes,
wrapped in the scars of crumbling walls,
where each careless brick laid,
was only more battlement to fall.
Amongst these remnants,
we've each cast our stones.
Now the true foundation
weeps within the wreckage,
as withered as the willows grown.
Could these lines have been foretold in the blueprints of the seeds,
somehow in the roots,
somehow in the branches of this tree.
Somewhere outside of heaven
an angel weeps.

Does an angel bleed?
Do all angels hinge upon wings?
I know not, I just know how I defined an angel to me.

Do all angels appear in visions or dreams?
I only know my angel gave their life to me.

I've seen ghosts in the eyes of an angel, just like me,
I've seen an angel weep.
I was there when an angel lost her wings.
I was there to hold her shuddering shoulders,
there to hold the weight of the weighted when they could no longer fly.
I picked up the shattered pieces as they in turn held me.
By what name do we call an angel?
Seraph… guardian… spirit?
I always just called my angel… mom.

Wish

I wish I had the hands to fix you
instead of just the endpoints of an embrace.
I know you see only the sorrows,
but I still see my angel's face.
I wish I could tuck you in
like that daydream little boy
and tell you it'll all be okay.
The words escape me in the face of it,
this sickness that tries to steal our light away,
but I still see my angel,
I still see the wings despite the fading trace.
I will never leave you momma
even as the twilight settles in.
You'll always be the brightest star,
just as on every horizon for me you've always been.
You'll always be the comfort of joy,
what was for me always the beginning and the end.
If only I could stitch your wings,
but my selfish feeble human hands would be afraid
that you'd only fly to the heavens
where jealous gods await.
I wish I could wrest the shadows that've plagued both you and I,
but I see the daylight fading through every tear that soaks my
eyes.

Echoes Amongst the Rain

Pages catch fire
from the sparks of syllables
sprung from the arson of my soul
as the urn of cellular vessels and synaptic webs
burn away
leaving only the ash of what remains
on the winds gone away
to plead echoes amongst the rain.

Watershed

Where do my tears have to go
when fallen wings have wrenched
the very depth of a heart?
With whom do I speak?
You who listens without hearing?
You who scream to drown the whole world?
You who never understood the weight of words?
I've heard time is like a river.
I've lost count of the drops that've flowed.
They've never made it to the silence,
but I've never known quite where they go.
What's it like to have a shoulder to absorb that acidic volume?
I've only this singular canvas that stretches from bone to bone.
Maybe if they all gathered at some distant horizon,
like the edges of a sea,
I could once again find a place
where the baptism of all the lost
could finally save an angel's son
never meant to be.

The Strength Within a Tear

The nimbus twilight slowly drifts across the horizon
as the daylight slowly fades.
I've often sat beside a window softly tapping
and admired the beauty of the gray.
I've always lived beside the waters
that impregnate the skies with their promises of tomorrow
and the deepest hues of spring.
I often watched the trails of raindrops upon
my reflection in the glass.
Sometimes I've walked within the tempest
and turned my face toward the canopy dismayed.

I'd wipe the raindrops from my eyes
and wonder at the weakness of the rain.
I'd often wonder how I was so broken
not to keep them inside.
I wondered at the echoes in the silence
of a thousand bricks aligned
along the rain shadow of a mountain
I was told the strong never climbed.
I've sat upon the cliffs and heard whispers in the wind,
only to see the barren foothills and empty canyons
that the shadows wander in.
One day I finally saw the illusion of those shadows
within the arid eyes of ghosts.
It was there, again descending,
beyond the shadow from which the desiccated feared to climb,
that I first saw the beauty of the hues within the gray.
I finally washed the illusion of the broken with the rain that fell
that day.

I often sit beside a window softly tapping
and admire the beauty of the gray.
I've always lived beside the waters
that impregnate the skies with their promises of tomorrow
and the deepest hues of spring.

I often watch the trails of rainfall upon
my reflection in the glass.
Sometimes I walk within the tempest
and turn my face toward the canopy unrestrained.

Here and There

Under clouded moonlight sky I realize
I can never separate myself from me.
Echoes still float upon the air and scatter in the breeze.
The same songs still strike the same tender chords.
The same tears still frame the same grin.

Reflection

If I could reach into your dreams,
replicate every nuance,
extract every gleam,
then perhaps I could be the person
you had always wanted me to be,
but in the mirror upon waking
I've always seen only me.
The shadow of that look
has haunted countless reflections
and threaded every patch
from time immemorial,
or at least as long as my own memory lasts.
I could cloak myself in expectations,
adorn my courtly mask…
the unwitting entertainer,
the jester,
the fire eater that burns within.
My mind is a prison,
my thoughts with no parole.
My mind is a singularity
with the gravity of a black hole.
I have dissected every adjective,
their nuances and their sounds.
I have thought about thinking
enough to know that I am.
A fish with a snorkel,
birthed in mercurial seas.
How profound a simple card could be,
framed by the love of another,
never quite knowing the turbulence,
the degree…
the longitude and latitude
of the wreckage along the shallow reef.
I've long gazed upon starlight from dunes far below,
only to wonder at the edges,
far from the tidal ebb and flow.

I’ve dived the depths for treasure
only for more questions to be found.
I’ve greeted waking moments
wondering how to make it through.
I’ve contemplated each present
into a chain of pasts…
like ink on paper that just bleeds through,
blurring evermore
the lines between strains of thought
and the distinctions between the hues.
I was born an alien from forgotten shores,
deciphering the hieroglyphics upon your walls,
listening to a drumbeat along paths I’ve walked alone,
stuck somewhere between futility
and a shadow of hope that brings me back
to the same saturated sky
and the same asphalt cracks.

Descending

From where have you descended,
you amalgams
(blood, feathers, bones
(bones as fragile and as strong
as the flow of the untamable gaseous sea))?
If I could only ask
I would ask if I might borrow your wings,
to know what you know,
to see what you've seen,
to know if perhaps your simple heart
is somehow more free.

Not To Wonder

I sit and stare at silken strands
woven upon an aging woodwork…
upon the midnight glass…
beside the trees…
under the crystal canopy…
surrounded by all that seems to pass…
each crumbling leaf…
every blade of grass…
we too shall pass.
I sit and wonder that you weave…
not to wonder, but just to weave.

Weighed by the same gravity you and I…
both subject to the same elements you and I…
both mortal just the same…
both getting by within this storm,
through the sunshine and the rain.
Yet, this heavy heart have you not,
this cauldron of joys and pain.
So, I sit and wonder as you weave…
not to wonder, but just to weave.

Dreaming To Fly

What force guides you to that light you see?
Is it that same impulse that I feel within me?
What do you hope to find?
It seems futile your flight,
seeking, lost… amongst so many lights.
You scorn the canopy for the lamp.
Is the starlight too high?
Have they ever shined in your eyes as they do in mine?
Have you ever looked beyond the streetlights,
beyond the delusions to which we both fly?
Are we both just seeking some mirage in the sky,
both of us doomed… only dreaming to fly.

Starlight

These same stars I gaze upon
for this fleeting speck of time
are those same stars that shined so bright on youth
I was then too innocent to know.
These same unfeeling lights
have been steadfast witnesses
to my joys, my sorrows, and everything in between.
Their waves echo back through the thin veil of time.
I think about those wishes on those stars and realize
that just like me those stars are different and yet I contemplate
what remains.
Shadows of regrets still linger beneath these same trees,
haunting the corners of my reality.
These trees will wither as to dust I turn
and these stars won't remember me
as their light fades before the vastness of the deep.
Let these cold lights burn out.
Let these shadowy trees wither away.
Let me not remember as time remembers me.

Meditation

I close my eyes, breathe out slow.
I try to stop within this moment,
but this moment gets lost in the flow.

In a mind bent on chaos,
stillness is an abstract ever distant shore.
Rivers of thought run defiantly free,
turning to rapids, and falling away
into the caverns of yesterday.

I close my eyes, breathe out very slow.
I try to stop within this moment,
but this moment within the current won't slow.

In seeking peace, rest is rarely found.
The faint pigments of impression framed by time
swirl within a synaptic expanse,
drowning the infinite within the mold of flesh and bone.

Inside Out

Cut through the skin.
The shroud comes undone.
Within the rhythmic chambers
flow secrets untold.
Fibrous thread stitches tapestries born of nothing,
slowly nursed by time.
The patchwork of protein
writhes on calcium sticks.
It is a capsule full of
stomach, liver, and intestinal worm.
Therein beats the heart,
that drips from this pen,
that draws from the inkwell
buried deep within.

Scribe

I've played poetry
with the bones
of skeletons
I've nursed within my skin.
I've silenced the din with scripted shadows,
when my stomach tightens,
when the waters rise,
and their familiar dance begins.
Their pleading is the only echo
in those lonely hours
when blue skies drain to gray.
With every note reflexively etched
upon page, after page, after page,
I've let creak
long rusted hinges
and let the voices have their say.
They talk to me of tomorrows,
of things only imagined
in restless moments
spent beneath sunset stars,
and of the calcium links
to the things that weigh
the steps before me.
They are the things
never left along the way
and it seems they will never
have naught to say,
upon these shredded forests
and the sands inexorable wake.

Profane

I’ve been to a sacred place
beyond the spaces within the stars
and yet as close as the profanity
within the depths of every bar.

One must journey past there and here,
past tides and fields.
One must lose their reflection in still waters…
watch the seas of sand stand still in the wind…
watch the white light
break within the faint glow of the rising western sun…
amidst the eastern hues of red bleeding into yellow,
shading citrus skies.

The World Still Lingers

The road still calls back
to that one upon which we used to play
when streetlights mattered,
when memories were barely made,
when one could only see puddles in the rain.
The leaves still change their hues,
each in their own way,
from chlorophyl to collage,
and still the seasons fade.
Birds still float upon the canopy.
Stars still sew the night.
The world still lingers and yet,
nothing is the same.

Western Horizons

This city is a city of memory,
of ghosts,
a kaleidoscopic landscape
of flowing concrete, passing faces,
outlined by sand and sea.
Every street is a frame to a movie reel,
filmed in fading light.
The child since forgotten,
save the impressions upon
a weighted heart,
plays before the mirror
alongside all the things
I had imagined myself to be.
This city's streets are paved with the powdered
shards of colored glass.
With the vestigial chambers
of carven chest,
I breathe unto thee,
my labored breath.
I take my leave of you,
my seaside alleyways,
my ghosts of fading light.
Perhaps I'll see the stars again
once wayward steps lead west.
I say goodbye to thee my city,
for with the last pieces of a glued heart rebroken,
I make thee a lasting tomb,
a mausoleum of all the things that were and should never have been,
of all the things that never will be
I long not to think of again.

Reverse Horizons

The intersections I crossed…
The streets I've walked…
All the stars that have passed
beneath a breadth of land…
salted of so many seas
and still the coast calls to me.
Summer days of triple A…
Moonlight boardwalks
and winter rains…
I remember liquor shots
drank with reckless thoughts
of futures never born.
I remember refuge sunsets
and the wasted joy of daydreams.
I remember all the ghosts
of all the heartaches and the pains.
I haven't forgotten every angel
that carved their piece of me.
I've never forgotten the emptiness of the glance
bestowed upon the battlefield of tattered seams.
But the sands still call,
the tide's ripple still sings,
of a place I remember
that once was so much…
a place where princes once imagined themselves kings.
But kingdoms are within
built with the scars of dusty tomes.
The skeletons all rattle
cadences of home,
where ghosts whispered hopes
like sirens upon restless seas…
where every wayward step
tried so hard to lay to rest
every splintered bone.
A friend once told me
that what was him

is not what he is now.
I’ll never forget that photo of three.
Each of us bare seasons
but I’ll never forget the stars,
the ones I hoped for, the ones gone by,
the ones I may have only imagined that I’d seen.
I'll never forget the murmur of the tide
upon scattered dunes…
the last light of twilight
upon the wetlands of home…
any more than I'll forget
the last words spoken
to turn what may have once been a heart
to the weight of stone.
I remember bottled messages
and starlight swings.
I remember high school promises
when I believed forever was real,
but every tapestry ever woven unraveled
with blades edge revealed.
I return to that sunset,
to those dunes,
and that rain… something forever changed.

Four Stops 'til Home

So many miles,
just four stops 'til home.
So many roads
my tired soul has roamed.
Here or there,
the weathered dunes still flow
and the windswept tides still foam.

The steps I've walked
don't fit the frame of miles.
They're within the stained-glass windows
through which I've seen horizons fade.
They're within the scar of smiles,
stitched with time's illusion
and woven along the way.

So many miles,
just four stops 'til home.
So many roads
my tired soul has roamed.
Here or there,
the weathered dunes still flow
and the windswept tides still foam.

Somewhere under shooting stars cast over swords of steel,
I rediscovered a wayward wanderer
all the whisperers had never known.
I remembered the flames of every passion
where suns had never set.
I remember every fleeting joy
and still cringe at every misstep.
Looking upon the road behind,
scattered with portents past,
I recall the tatters of promises that began with forgotten breaths.

So many miles,

just four stops ‘til home.
So many roads
my tired soul has roamed.
Here or there,
the weathered dunes still flow
and the windswept tides still foam.

Bring me no horizon,
for the farthest journeys
are not always measured
within the limits of miles.
Not all depths can be measured
with the weight of stone.

So many miles,
just four stops ‘til home.
So many roads
my tired soul has roamed.
Here or there,
the weathered dunes still flow
and the windswept tides still foam.

I am an immigrant of paradox
between a then and now.
I am a transplant from there not here
and yet inevitably here and now.
I am the heir of tragic kingdoms,
of both the masses and the lost.
I scratch words within haunted forests
to both remember and forget
where these steps have wandered
along this wooded path.

So many miles,
just four stops ‘til home.
So many roads
my tired soul has roamed.
Here or there,

the weathered dunes still flow
and the windswept tides still foam.

Within the Fading Light

It's been a season…
of reflection,
of acceptance,
of… regrets,
and the remembrance of the rain.
Though it falls so seldom here
it's never left
the echoes of the steady rhythm
etched upon my brain.
Within the vastness of the currents,
all the rivers run just the same.
We can travel a thousand light years
and never leave the reflections and refractions
imprinted upon the panes along the way.
I remain the patchwork of ungentle hands
and someone else's broken dreams,
the unnamed creature of monstrous lore,
with just a few more stitches to my name.
I'd light the script of a thousand suns
if only to find the promise of a quiet sunset
along some final shore.
I've sought so many horizons,
throughout time and space alike,
but I've never found any answers within those fading lights.
I return to the dawn of my seeking,
just to transcribe these coded lines again.
Therein lies the only peace I've ever truly known,
within the resin of these pages,
filled with the meditation of a pen.

About the Author

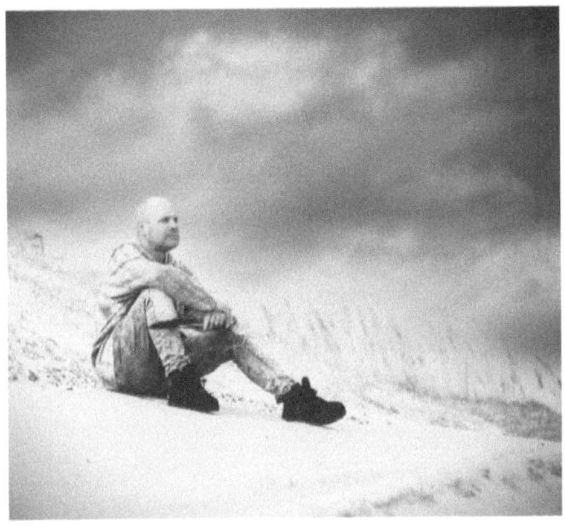

[Photograph by Cody Snyder]

Born in a seaside city, inspired by coastal sunsets and drifting dunes, I began writing poetry in my youth and coloring my words with the world I grew up in, full of brackish waters, tidal wetlands, and roving shore birds. An awkward kid who eagerly awaited the next book fair, I grew up immersing myself in worlds of myth and magic, traversing stars, and finding refuge in dusty shelves of lore.

As the years have passed, I have never forgotten my original passion. Whether art, music, stories, or poetry, creativity is born from the spark of humanity which ultimately connects us all. It is a vehicle through which we can each find our voice. My work delves into many aspects of mental health, from anxiety to depression, as well as discussing family and the intricacies of interpersonal relationships. Through writing and poetry, I overcame my early struggles and found my own voice. With that voice I hope to share the value that can be found in creative expression and resonate with those that may be going through mental health challenges of their own.

www.ingramcontent.com/pod-product-compliance
Ingram Content Group UK Ltd.
Pitfield, Milton Keynes, MK11 3LW, UK
UKHW041632190726
13854UKWH00006B/2460

9 781304 072672